# MONKEYPOX VIRUS

## :How monkeypox spread, prevention, vaccine and how to protect the children

**By**

**Dr.Alex Woodrow**

# Table of contents

INTRODUCTION

What is monkeypox

Is monkeypox destructive

When would it be a good idea for someone to gets tested for monkeypox?

Monkeypox side effects

How does monkeypox spread

What are the well-known ways kids might get monkeypox?

How could guardians shield their children from monkeypox?

The most effective method to forestall monkeypox

Antibody security

How could an individual lower the possibility of getting monkeypox at places like raves, gatherings, clubs, and celebrations?

Bug and monkeypox

Treatment

UNITED STATE flare-up 2022 circumstance synopsis

What clinical  experts ought to be aware

Interval Clinical Guidance for the Treatment of Monkeypox

Clinical Countermeasures Available for the Treatment of Monkeypox

CONCLUSION

# INTRODUCTION

## What is monkeypox

Monkeypox is an uncommon illness brought about by disease with the monkeypox infection. Monkeypox infection is important for a similar group of infections as variola infection, the infection that causes smallpox. Monkeypox side effects are like smallpox side effects, yet milder, and monkeypox is seldom lethal. Monkeypox isn't connected with chickenpox.

Monkeypox was found in 1958 when two flare-ups of a pox-like illness happened in states of monkeys saved for research. Notwithstanding being named "monkeypox," the wellspring of the illness stays obscure. Notwithstanding, African rodents and non-human primates (like monkeys) could hold onto the infection and taint individuals.

The principal human instance of monkeypox was kept in 1970. Preceding the 2022 episode, monkeypox had been accounted for in individuals in a few focal and western African nations. Already, practically all monkeypox cases in individuals beyond Africa were connected to worldwide travel to nations where the illness usually happens or through imported creatures. These cases happened on different mainlands.

Sorts of monkeypox

There are two sorts of monkeypox infection:

•West African and

• Congo Basin.

Contaminations in the ongoing flare-up are from the West African sort.

# Is monkeypox destructive

Contaminations with the kind of monkeypox infection recognized in this flare-up — the West African sort — are seldom lethal. More than the vast majority of individuals who get this type of infection are probably going to make due. Be that as it may, individuals with debilitated invulnerable frameworks, youngsters under 8 years old, individuals with a background marked by dermatitis, and individuals who are pregnant or breastfeeding might be bound to get genuinely sick or pass on.

The Congo Basin kind of monkeypox infection has a casualty rate of around 10%.

# When would it be a good idea for someone to gets tested for monkeypox?

Individuals who think they have monkeypox or have had close private contact with somebody who has monkeypox ought to visit a medical care supplier to assist them with choosing if they should be tried for monkeypox. Assuming that they conclude that you ought to be tried, they will work with you to gather the examples and send them to a research facility for testing

# Monkeypox side effects

Individuals with monkeypox get a rash that might be situated on or close to the privates (penis, gonads, labia, and vagina) or rear-end (butthole) and could be on different regions like the hands, feet, chest, face, or mouth.

The rash will go through a few

phases, including scabs, before mending.

The rash can at first seem to be pimples or rankles and might be agonizing or irritated.

**Different side effects of monkeypox can include:**

Fever

Chills

Enlarged lymph hubs

Fatigue

Muscle throbs and spinal pain

Cerebral pain

Respiratory side effects (for example sore throat, nasal clog, or hack)

You might encounter all or a couple of side effects

Once in a while, individuals have influenza-like side effects before the rash.

Certain individuals get a rash first, trailed by different side effects.

Others just experience a rash.

**How long do monkeypox side effects last?**

Monkeypox side effects ordinarily start somewhere around 3 weeks of openness to the infection. On the off chance that somebody has influenza-like

side effects, they will generally foster a rash 1 after 4 days.

**How would it be advisable for me if I noticed I have a side effect of monkeypox?**

See a medical care supplier on the off chance that you notice a new or unexplained rash or other monkeypox side effects.

Remind the medical care supplier that monkeypox is available in the United States.

Keep away from close contact (counting private actual contact) with others until you see a medical services supplier.

Stay away from close contact with pets or different creatures until you see a medical care supplier.

On the off chance that you're sitting tight for test results, follow similar safety measures.

If your experimental outcome is positive, remain segregated and notice another counteraction rehearses until your rash has mended, all scabs have tumbled off, and a new layer of flawless skin has framed.

Stay confined on the off chance that you have a fever, sore throat, nasal blockage, or hack. Simply go out to see a medical services supplier or for a crisis. Keep away from public transportation.

On the off chance that you should leave seclusion, cover the rash and wear a well-fitting veil.

# How does monkeypox spread

Monkeypox can be spread from the time side effects start until the rash has recuperated, all scabs have tumbled off, and a new layer of skin has been shaped. The disease normally endures to a month.

If by chance that You Have a recently or Unexplained Rash or Other Symptoms.

Keep away from close contact, including sex or getting physically involved with anybody, until you have been looked at by a medical services supplier.

If you don't have a supplier or medical coverage, visit a general wellbeing facility close to you.

At the point when you see a medical services supplier, wear a veil, and advise them that this infection is flowing nearby.

**Monkeypox spreads in a couple of ways which include :**

Monkeypox can spread to anybody through close, individual, frequently skin-to-skin contact, including:

Direct contact with monkeypox rash, scabs, or body liquids from an individual with monkeypox.

Contacting objects, textures (attire, bedding, or towels), and surfaces that have been utilized by somebody with monkeypox.

Contact with respiratory emissions.

This immediate contact can occur during private contact, including:

Oral, butt-centric, and vaginal sex or contacting the privates (penis, balls, labia, and vagina) or rear-end (butthole) of an individual with monkeypox.

Embracing, back rub and kissing.

Drawn out an eye to eye contact.

Contacting textures and items during sex that were utilized by an individual with monkeypox for example, bedding, towels, obsession stuff, and sex toys.

A pregnant woma can infect their baby with the virus through the placenta.

It's likewise workable for individuals to get monkeypox from tainted creatures, either by being damaged or chomped by the creature or by planning or eating meat or utilizing items from a contaminated creature.

An individual with monkeypox can spread it to others from the time side effects start until the rash has completely mended and a new layer of skin has been shaped. The ailment ordinarily endures to a month.

On the off chance that the infection can be spread when somebody has no side effects.

How frequently monkeypox is spread through respiratory emissions, or when an individual with monkeypox side effects may be bound to spread the infection through respiratory discharges.

Whether monkeypox can be spread through semen, vaginal liquids, pee, or defecation.

**Find the accompanying ways to forestall getting monkeypox:**

**Deal with yourself**

Stay away from close, skin-to-skin contact with individuals who have a rash that looks like monkeypox.

Try not to touch or get in contact with the rash or scabs of a person with monkeypox.

Try not have close relationship like sex or hug with someone with monkeypox

Keep away from contact with items and materials that an individual with monkeypox has utilized.

Try not to use or hold eating utensils or house material that an individual with monkeypox have used.

Try not to deal with or use the bed material, towels, or dress of an individual with monkeypox.

Clean up frequently with a cleanser and water or utilize a liquor-based hand sanitizer, particularly before eating or contacting your face and after you utilize the washroom.

In Central and West Africa, keep away from contact with creatures that can spread monkeypox infection, typically rodents and primates. Likewise, stay away from debilitated or dead creatures, as well as bedding or different materials they have contacted

Immunization

CDC suggests immunization for individuals who have been presented with monkeypox and individuals who might be bound to get monkeypox.

# What are the well-known ways kids might get monkeypox?

"Monkeypox can be spreads through close skin-to-skin contact with an individual with it, which, on account of youngsters, could incorporate holding, snuggling, taking care of, as well as through shared towels, bedding, cups, and utensils, the sickness can likewise be communicated to a hatchling during pregnancy or to an infant through close contact during and after birth.

infection can persevere on surfaces, and those living with somebody who has monkeypox should be cautious with bedding and different materials on which the infection could endure. It is proposed that all possibly tainted sheet material, towels, and attire be washed thoroughly and put through the dryer.

It's truly critical to perceive that there have just been a couple of affirmed cases in kids up until this point, and the vast majority of those youngsters had been in close contact with a known monkeypox case, the most probable situation for youngsters to get monkeypox is through supported family openness. "a dad, a mother, a youthful grown-up or high schooler with monkeypox in the home," "Very much like smallpox, it tends to be spread through respiratory drops and pollution of surfaces, however, it isn't quite so infectious as smallpox.

**How does monkeypox influence youngsters?**

The children who are at most noteworthy danger for extreme sickness are the people who are under age 8, "They usually more often than not experience difficulties like pneumonia and mind aggravation. The actual bruises can become tainted and cause cellulitis and sepsis. The explanation kids are bound to foster cellulitis as well as sepsis is that more youthful youngsters make some harder memories not scratching the injuries."

The injuries are frequently very excruciating, "They can be difficult to such an extent that individuals once in a while need long-term administration of agony, "In kids that turns into a genuine and grievous test for us."

The sickness may not be as dangerous as HIV, however, no one needs to encounter that degree of agony, Moreover, it can cause critical scarring. "Take a gander at the more seasoned pictures of individuals who had smallpox. "The vast majority would need to stay away from those scars."

Both the monkeypox immunization and an exploratory treatment called TPOXX are presently accessible for youngsters under unique extended admittance conventions.

# How could guardians shield their children from monkeypox?

"The main thing guardians can do to safeguard their kids is to ensure they don't get monkeypox, "That might mean keeping away from specific exercises that place them at high danger and avoiding potential risks they in any case probably won't take.

**Individuals bound to get monkeypox include:**

Individuals who have been recognized by group of people as a contact of somebody with monkeypox

Individuals who know that one of their sexual partners within fourteen days has been determined to have monkeypox

Individuals who had numerous sexual accomplices in the beyond 2 weeks in a space with known monkeypox

Individuals whose thier status or work might open them to the exposure of the virus, for example,

Research facility laborers who perform testing for orthopoxviruses
Research facility laborers who handle societies or creatures with orthopoxviruses
Some assigned medical care or general well-being laborers

# The most effective method to forestall monkeypox

## Antibody security

The favored immunization to safeguard against monkeypox is JYNNEOS, which is a two-portion antibody. It requires 14 days after getting the second portion of JYNNEOS for its insusceptible security to arrive at its most extreme.

The ACAM2000 anti virus might be an option in place of JYNNEOS. ACAM2000 is a solitary portion immunization, and it requires a month after inoculation for its resistant insurance to arrive at its greatest. Notwithstanding, it has the potential for additional secondary effects and antagonistic

occasions than JYNNEOS. It isn't suggested for individuals with seriously debilitated insusceptible frameworks and a few different circumstances.
Individuals ought to play it safe to diminish their openness to monkeypox until insusceptible insurance from immunizations has arrived at its most extreme. Counsel your medical services supplier to check whether you ought to get immunization against monkeypox and if you ought to get ACAM2000 rather than JYNNEOS.

## More secure sex and party

While CDC attempts to contain the current monkeypox episode and more deeply study the infection, this data can assist you with pursuing informed decisions when you are in circumstances or where monkeypox could be spread. Monkeypox isn't viewed as a physically sent illness, yet it is many times communicated through close, supported actual contact, which can incorporate sexual contact.

## How might an individual lower their risk during sex?

Make a propensity for trading contact data with any new accomplice to take into consideration sexual wellbeing follow-up, if necessary.

Talk with your accomplice about any monkeypox side effects and know about any new or unexplained rash or sore on both of your bodies, including the mouth, private parts (penis, gonads, vulva, or vagina), or rear-end (butthole). If you or your accomplice has or as of late had monkeypox side effects, or you have a new or unexplained rash anyplace on your body, don't engage in sexual relations and see a medical services supplier. Now and again, side effects might be gentle, and certain individuals may not realize they have monkeypox.

On the off chance that you or an accomplice has monkeypox or figure you might have monkeypox, the most effective way to safeguard yourself as well as other people is to keep away from sex of any sort (oral, butt-centric, vaginal) and kissing or contacting each other's bodies — while you are wiped out. Particularly try not to contact any impulsive.

Try not to share things like towels, or personal belongings like toothbrush,comb.

Regardless of whether you feel great, here are far to decrease your possibilities of being presented with monkeypox assuming you are physically dynamic:

Enjoy some time off from exercises that increment openness to monkeypox until you are fourteen days after your subsequent portion. This will significantly lessen your risk .

Limit your number of sex accomplices to decrease your probability of openness.

Spaces like reserved alcoves, saunas, sex clubs, or private and public sex parties, where personal, frequently mysterious sexual contact with different accomplices happens — are bound to spread monkeypox.

Condoms (plastic or polyurethane) may safeguard your rear-end (butthole), mouth, penis, or vagina from openness to monkeypox. Nonetheless, condoms alone may not forestall all openings to monkeypox since the rash can happen on different pieces of the body.

Gloves (plastic, polyurethane, or nitrile) could likewise decrease the chance of openness if embedding fingers or hands into the vagina or the rear end. The gloves should cover all uncovered skin and be eliminated cautiously to try not to contact the external surface.

Try not to kiss or trade spit since monkeypox can spread along these lines.

Stroke off together a ways off without contacting one another and without contacting any ill-advised.
Have virtual sex with no face-to-face contact.
Consider engaging in sexual relations with your garments on or covering regions where the rash is available, decreasing however much skin-to-skin contact as could reasonably be expected.
Cowhide or plastic stuff likewise gives an obstruction to skin-to-skin contact; simply make certain to change or clean garments/gear among accomplices and after use.
Know that monkeypox can likewise spread through respiratory discharges with close, eye-to-eye contact.
Make sure to clean up, fixation gear, sex toys, and any textures (bedding, towels, garments) after having intercourse.

**How should an individual be responsible if they have a new or unexplained rash or different side effects?**

Try not to have sex or get physically involved with anybody until you have been looked at by a medical care supplier.

If you don't have a supplier or medical coverage, visit a general wellbeing center close to you.

At the point when you see a medical care supplier, wear a cover, and advise them that this infection is circling nearby.

Stay away from get-togethers, particularly assuming that they include close, individual, skin-to-skin contact.

Ponder individuals you have had close, individual, or sexual contact with during the most recent 21 days, including individuals you met through dating applications. To assist with halting the spread, you may be inquired as to whether you have gotten a monkeypox.

# How could an individual lower the possibility of getting monkeypox at places like raves, gatherings, clubs, and celebrations?

While pondering what to do, search out data from believed sources like the nearby wellbeing division. Second, consider how much close, individual, skin-to-skin contact is probably going to happen on the occasion you intend to join in. On the off chance that you feel wiped out or have a rash, go to no social event, and see a medical services supplier.

Celebrations, occasions, and shows where participants are completely dressed and improbable to share skin-to-skin contact are more secure. In any case, participants ought to be aware of exercises (like kissing) that could spread monkeypox.

A rave, party, or club where there is insignificant clothing and where there is immediate, individual, frequently skin-to-skin contact has some risk. Keep away from any ill-advised you see in others and consider limiting skin-to-skin contact.

Encased spaces, for example, reserved alcoves, saunas, sex clubs, or private and public sex parties where personal, frequently mysterious sexual contact with numerous accomplices happens, may have a higher probability of spreading monkeypox.

**Assemble settings**

Monkeypox is an illness that can cause influenza-like side effects and a rash. Human-to-human transmission of monkeypox infection happens by direct contact with injuries or contaminated body liquids, or from openness to respiratory discharges during delayed eye-to-eye contact. An individual is viewed as irresistible until there is full recuperating of the rash with the development of a new layer of skin.

If a staff part, volunteer, or occupant of a gathered living setting has a monkeypox infection disease, transmission could happen inside the setting. Assemble residing settings are offices or other lodgings where individuals who are not related dwell in nearness and offer somewhere around one well-known room (e.g., dozing room, kitchen, washroom, parlor). Gather residing settings can incorporate restorative and detainment offices, destitute sanctuaries, bunch homes, quarters at organizations of advanced education, part-time employee lodging, private substance use treatment offices, and other comparable settings. These settings might give individual consideration benefits however are not customary medical services settings (for example clinics). Assuming that medical care administrations are given nearby, they are normally given in unambiguous medical care regions or by outside medical services faculty (e.g., home medical services laborers). In these conditions, medical care staff ought to follow proposals in Infection Control.

**If a monkeypox case has been recognized in a gathered living office, think about the accompanying activities:**

Speak with staff, volunteers, and inhabitants — Provide clear data to staff, volunteers, and occupants about monkeypox counteraction, including the potential for transmission through close, supported actual contact, including sexual activity. Give anticipation direction including contemplations to more secure sex. Keep messages reality-based to abstain from presenting shame while conveying about monkeypox.

**Answer cases — Consider the accompanying activities to answer cases in the office:**

Test and medicinally assess staff, volunteers, or inhabitants who are thought to have monkeypox. In a perfect world, individuals distinguished to have monkeypox will stay separated away from others until there is full mending of the rash with the development of a new layer of skin, which ordinarily requires two to about a month.

Counsel your state, ancestral, nearby, or regional wellbeing division before suspending disengagement.

Guarantee that inhabitants with monkeypox wear a well-fitting dispensable veil over their nose and mouth and cover any skin injuries with long jeans and long sleeves, swathes, or a sheet or outfit if they need to leave the disconnection region or on the other hand, if separation regions are not yet accessible.

Some assemble living offices might have the option to give segregation on location while others might have to get inhabitants off-site to disconnect. Occupant detachment spaces ought to have an entryway that can be shut down and a committed washroom that different inhabitants don't utilize. Different occupants who test positive for monkeypox can remain in a similar room.

Disconnect staff or volunteers who have monkeypox away from gather settings until they are completely recuperated. Adaptable, non-corrective wiped-out leave arrangements for staff individuals are basic to forestall the spread of monkeypox.
Diminish the quantity of staff who are entering the seclusion regions to staff who are crucial for segregation region activities.
Oversee squander from confinement regions (i.e., dealing with, stockpiling, treatment, and removal of ruined PPE, patient dressings, and so forth).
Required squander the board practices and class assignment can vary contingent upon the Monkeypox infection clade (strain) the patient has. Cases in the ongoing episode have been recognized to be West African clade, and waste from these patients is named directed clinical waste (Category B). Offices ought to likewise conform to state and nearby guidelines for dealing with, stockpiling, treatment, and removal of waste.
Recognize individuals who could have been presented with monkeypox — Facilities ought to work with their state, ancestral, nearby screen the soundness of any staff, volunteers, or inhabitants who could have had close contact with somebody who has monkeypox. Contact following can assist

with distinguishing individuals with openness and assist with forestalling extra cases. Be that as it may, this probably won't be attainable in all settings.

Use openness risk evaluation suggestions to distinguish individuals who had a serious level of openness to somebody with monkeypox, where conceivable. The state, ancestral, neighborhood, or regional wellbeing office can give present openness inoculation on individuals with serious level openings.

In offices where contact following isn't practical, staff, volunteers, and occupants who invested energy in a similar region as somebody with monkeypox ought to be considered to have a moderate or low level of openness, contingent upon the qualities of the setting (for example level of swarming). Post-openness immunization isn't required for low or moderate degree openings except if considered proper by the state or nearby wellbeing division.

Guarantee admittance to handwashing — Soap and water or hand sanitizer with something like 60% liquor ought to be accessible consistently and at no expense to all staff, volunteers, and occupants. Any individual who contacts sores or apparel, materials, or surfaces that might have had contact with injuries ought to clean up right away.

Clean and sanitize the regions where individuals with monkeypox invested energy — Avoid exercises that could spread dried material from sores (e.g., utilization of fans, dry tidying, clearing, or vacuuming).. Perform sanitization utilizing an EPA-enlisted sanitizer with an Emerging Viral Pathogens guarantee, which might be tracked down on EPA's List Q. Follow the producer's bearings for focus, contact time,  care,and dealing with. Materials can be washed utilizing a customary cleanser and warm water. Dirtied clothing ought to be delicately and immediately contained in a clothing pack and never be shaken or dealt with in a way that might scatter irresistible material. Covering beddings in confinement regions (for example with sheets, covers, or a plastic cover) can work with simpler washing.

Give proper individual defensive gear (PPE) for staff, volunteers, and inhabitants — Employers are answerable for guaranteeing that specialists are safeguarded from openness to Monkeypox infection and that laborers are not presented to hurtful degrees of synthetics utilized for cleaning and sterilization. PPE ought to be worn by staff, volunteers, or occupants in these conditions:

Entering confinement regions — Staff who enter seclusion regions ought to wear an outfit, gloves, eye security, and a NIOSH-supported particulate respirator furnished with N95 channels or higher.
Clothing — When taking care of grimy clothing from individuals with known or thought monkeypox contamination, staff, volunteers, or occupants ought to wear an outfit, gloves, eye insurance, and a well-fitting veil or respirator. PPE isn't required after the wash cycle is finished.
Cleaning and sterilization — Staff, volunteers, or occupants ought to wear an outfit, gloves, eye security, and a well-fitting veil or respirator while cleaning regions where individuals with monkeypox invested energy.
Managers should follow OSHA's principles on Bloodborne Pathogens Respiratory Protection, and different prerequisites, including those laid out by state plans, at whatever point such necessities apply.

**Home sanitizer**

Reason for Home Disinfection

Individuals with monkeypox who don't need hospitalization might be segregated at home. Monkeypox spreads between individuals through direct contact with an irresistible rash, body liquids, or by respiratory emissions during delayed, up close, and personal contact. Transmission of Monkeypox infection is conceivable from the beginning of the main side effects until the scabs have isolated and the skin has completely mended.

During the irresistible timeframe, body liquids, respiratory emissions, and injury material from individuals with monkeypox can debase the climate. Poxviruses can get by in materials, clothing, and on natural surfaces, especially when in dull, cool, and low dampness conditions. In one review, specialists found live infection 15 days after a patient's house was left empty. Concentrates on a show that other firmly related Orthopoxviruses can make due in a climate, like a family, for weeks or months. Permeable materials (bedding, clothing, and so on) may hold onto live infection for longer timeframes than non-permeable (plastic, glass, metal) surfaces.
Orthopoxviruses are exceptionally delicate to UV light. Regardless of the capacity of Orthopoxviruses to continue in the climate, they are likewise delicate

to numerous sanitizers, and sanitization is suggested for all areas (like home and vehicle) where an individual with monkeypox has invested energy, as well as, for things viewed as possibly defiled.

Sanitizer

**Utilize an EPA-enrolled sanitizer**, as per the producer's guidelines. Follow all producer headings for use, including focus, contact time,care and dealing with. While picking a sanitizer, it is essential to consider any potential wellbeing perils, and don't blend sanitizers or add different synthetics.

Follow these means for protected and powerful sanitizer use:

**Make sure that your item is EPA-enrolled:** Find the EPA enlistment number on the item.

Peruse the bearings: Follow the item's headings. Check "use locales" and "surface sorts" to ensure this is the right item for your surface. Then, read the "preparatory articulations."

Pre-clean the surface: Make sure to wash the surface with cleanser and water assuming the bearings notice pre-cleaning or on the other hand if the surface is grimy. Soil can hold the sanitizer back from working.

Follow the contact time: Follow the guidelines: The surface ought to stay wet for how much time is shown to guarantee the item is compelling. Reapply if fundamental.

**Cleaning and Disinfection**

During detachment at home, individuals with monkeypox should clean and sanitize the spaces they involve routinely to restrict family pollution.

Segregating ALONE IN HOME: People with monkeypox who are detaching alone at home ought to consistently spotless and sanitize the spaces they possess, including usually contacted surfaces and things, to restrict family defilement. Perform hand cleanliness subsequently utilizing a liquor-based hand rub (ABHR) that contains something like 60% liquor, or cleanser and water assuming ABHR is inaccessible.

Segregating WITH OTHERS IN HOME: People with monkeypox who are separated in a home from other people who don't have monkeypox ought to follow the seclusion and disease control direction, and any common spaces, machines, or things ought to be sanitized quickly following use.

Individuals who have recuperated from monkeypox and whose separation period has finished ought to direct careful sterilization of the relative multitude of spaces inside the home that they had been in touch with. Follow the means underneath to limit the chance of disease to others in your home after recuperation.

If cleaning and sterilization are finished by somebody other than the individual with monkeypox, that individual ought to wear, at least, expendable clinical gloves and a respirator or well-fitting veil.

Standard apparel that completely covers the skin ought to be worn, and afterward quickly washed by proposals underneath.

Hand cleanliness ought to be performed utilizing an ABHR, or cleanser and water assuming ABHR are inaccessible.

Center around sanitizing things and surfaces that were in direct contact with the skin of the individual with monkeypox, or frequently within the sight of the individual with monkeypox, during disconnection. If uncertain, clean.

Try not to dry residue or clear it as this might spread irresistible particles.

Wet cleaning strategies are favored like sanitizer wipes, splashes, and wiping.

Vacuuming is OK by utilizing a vacuum with a high-effectiveness air channel. If not accessible, guarantee the individual vacuuming wears a well-fitting cover or respirator.

Clean and sanitize family in the accompanying request:

**General waste regulation**

Gather and contain in a fixed sack any dirty waste, for example, gauzes, paper towels, food bundling, and other general garbage things.

Clothing

**Assemble** defiled apparel and materials before whatever else in the room is cleaned. Try not to shake the materials as this could spread irresistible particles.

Hard surfaces and family things

Upholstered furniture and another delicate outfitting

Rug and deck

Garbage removal

**Clothing**

Utilized or tainted attire, cloths and bedding materials, towels, and other texture things ought to be contained until washed. At the point when at all potential, individuals with monkeypox ought to deal with and wash their grimy clothing. Clothing ought not to be blended in with that of different individuals from the family.

**Follow these washing methods:**

Handle ruined clothing as per standard works, staying away from contact with defiles from the rash that might be available on the clothing.

Dirtied clothing ought to never be shaken or taken care of in a way that might spread irresistible particles.

In-home clothing offices:

Move ruined clothing things to be washed in an impermeable holder or sack that can be sanitized thereafter. On the other hand, a texture pack might be utilized that can likewise be washed alongside the dirty things.

Wash clothing in a standard clothes washer with a cleanser, adhering to mark guidelines. Clothing sanitizers might be utilized however are excessive.

**In-home clothing offices not accessible:**

At the point when in-home clothing offices (offices not imparted to different families) are not accessible, people ought to organize with their nearby general wellbeing division to decide on proper washing choices.

Hard Surfaces (and non-permeable vehicle insides)

Regularly perfect and sanitize normally contacted surfaces and things (like counters or light switches) utilizing an EPA-enrolled sanitizer as per the producer's directions.

This incorporates surfaces like tables, ledges, entryway handles, latrine flush handles, fixtures, light switches, and floors.

Incorporate inside surfaces of fridge, cooler, different machines, inside bureau spaces, or drawers assuming they have been gotten to by the individual with monkeypox.

Things and surfaces inside the home that have likely not been in touch with the individual while debilitated with monkeypox needn't bother with to be cleaned.

Attire and things for drawers or boxes that the poor person has been in touch with, or the immediate presence of the individual with monkeypox.

Wash dirtied dishes and eating utensils in a dishwasher with a cleanser and high temp water or by hand with boiling water and dish cleanser.

Upholstered Furniture, Carpet, and Soft Furnishing (and permeable vehicle insides)

On the off chance that the individual with monkeypox had direct skin contact as well as an extreme waste of liquids from rashes onto delicate decorations, like upholstered furniture, floor coverings, carpets, and sleeping cushions, steam cleaning can be thought of. Examine with state or nearby wellbeing experts for additional direction.

On the off chance that the individual with monkeypox had insignificant contact with delicate decorations, sanitize the surface with a surface-proper sanitizer.

**Garbage Disposal**

For the most part, the board of waste from homes, incorporating those of individuals with monkeypox secluding at home, ought to go on as should be expected. Civil waste administration frameworks regularly gather and discard squander materials from people with irresistible illnesses and can do so securely utilizing existing techniques.

The individual with monkeypox ought to utilize a committed, lined garbage bin in the room where they are secluded.

Any gloves, gauzes, or other waste and expendable things that have been in direct contact with skin ought to be set in a fixed plastic pack, then discarded in the committed garbage bin.

The individual with monkeypox or other family individuals ought to utilize gloves while eliminating trash containers and taking care of and discarding garbage.

Assuming proficient cleaning administrations are utilized, treat or potentially discard squander as per material state, neighborhood, ancestral, and regional regulations and guidelines for squandering the board.

# Bug and monkeypox

Contaminated creatures can spread Monkeypox infection to individuals, and potential individuals who are tainted can spread Monkeypox infection to creatures through close contact, including petting, snuggling, embracing, kissing, licking, sharing dozing regions, and sharing food.

Individuals with monkeypox ought to stay away from contact with creatures, including pets, homegrown creatures, and natural life to forestall the spreading of the infection. Assuming that your pet is presented with monkeypox:

Try not to give up, euthanize, or forsake pets as a result of an expected openness or Monkeypox infection

Try not to wipe or wash your pet with compound sanitizers, liquor, hydrogen peroxide, or different items, for example, hand sanitizer, counter-cleaning wipes, or other modern or surface cleaners.

If the individual with monkeypox didn't have close contact with pets after the side effect begins, ask companions or relatives who live in a different home to be the creature's overseer until the individual with monkeypox completely recuperates. Close contact incorporates petting, nestling, embracing, kissing, licking, sharing dozing regions, and sharing food.

After the individual with monkeypox is recuperated, sanitize your home before bringing sound creatures back; follow Disinfecting Home and Other Non-Healthcare Settings.

Pets that had close contact with an indicative individual with monkeypox ought to be kept at home and away from different creatures and individuals for 21 days after the latest contact. Tainted individuals shouldn't deal with uncovered pets. The individual with monkeypox ought to stay away from close contact with the uncovered creature, and whenever the situation allows, request that another family cares for the creature until the individual with monkeypox is completely recuperated.

At times, it could be important to detach and focus on creatures that have been presented with monkeypox in an area other than the home. For instance, individuals who are immunocompromised, pregnant, have small kids present (<8 years old), or with a background marked by atopic dermatitis or skin inflammation, shouldn't give care to creatures that had close contact with an individual with monkeypox as they might be at expanded risk for serious results from monkeypox illness.

Assuming you have monkeypox and should focus on your sound pets during home segregation, clean up, or utilize a liquor-based hand rub when focusing on them. It is likewise vital to cover any skin rash to the most ideal degree (for example long sleeves, long jeans), and wear gloves and a well-fitting cover or respirator while considering your creatures.

Try not to put a veil on your pet.

Keep away from close contact with your pet.

Guarantee your pet can't coincidentally come into contact with debased articles in the home like apparel, sheets, and towels utilized by the individual with monkeypox.

Try not to allow creatures to come into contact with rashes, swathes, and body liquids.

Guarantee food, toys, bedding, or different things that you accommodate your creature during its detachment don't come in that frame of mind with skin or uncovered rash.

## What to do if a pet gives indications of monkeypox

While we don't have the foggiest idea about every one of the side effects tainted creatures might have, watch the creature for expected indications of disease including torpidity, absence of hunger, hacking, nasal discharges, swelling, fever, or potentially pimple-or rankle like skin rash. Call your veterinarian on the off chance that you notice a creature seems debilitated in something like 21 days of having contact with a plausible or affirmed individual monkeypox. A veterinarian can assist with informing your state general wellbeing veterinarian or state creature wellbeing official.

Don't euthanize pets with thought monkeypox except if coordinated by a veterinarian.

Try not to wipe or wash your pet with substance sanitizers, liquor, hydrogen peroxide, or different items, for example, hand sanitizer, counter-cleaning wipes, or other modern or surface cleaners.

Moves toward taking on the off chance that you think your pet has monkeypox

Get your pet tried if they have had close contact with an individual with plausible or affirmed monkeypox and they have another rash or two other clinical signs. Call your veterinarian if you notice a creature seems debilitated in 21 days of having contact with a plausible or affirmed individual monkeypox. A veterinarian can assist with telling your state general wellbeing veterinarian or state creature wellbeing official.

Conceivable clinical indications of monkeypox in creatures incorporate laziness, absence of hunger, hacking, swelling, nasal as well as eye discharges or hull, fever, or potentially pox-like skin sores (may at first look like a pimple or rankle before movement to a trademark monkeypox sore) or rash.

Separate the debilitated pet or creature from different creatures and limit direct contact with individuals for something like 21 days after turning out to be sick or until completely recuperated.

It is desirable over to keep creatures with indications of disease secluded in their home and away from anybody who has not had monkeypox.

Individuals who are immunocompromised, pregnant, have small kids present (<8 years old), or with a background marked by atopic dermatitis or skin inflammation, shouldn't give care to sick creatures that had close contact with an individual with monkeypox.

Clean up frequently and utilize individual defensive hardware (PPE) while focusing on and tidying up after debilitated creatures. PPE incorporates wearing gloves, utilizing eye insurance (security glasses, goggles, or face safeguard), wearing a well-fitting cover or respirator (in a perfect world a dispensable NIOSH-supported N95 sifting facepiece respirator), and wearing an expendable outfit.

If an expendable outfit isn't accessible, wear clothing that completely covers the skin (for example long sleeves, or long jeans), and promptly take off and wash clothing after contact with the creature, creature nooks, or creature bedding.

Cautiously eliminate PPE to keep away from self-defilement.

Utilize a liquor-based hand rub or wash hands with a cleanser and water after PPE has been taken out.

Counsel your neighborhood general wellbeing division for rules for garbage removal, however, **broad precautionary measures include:**

Utilize a devoted, lined garbage bin for all possibly polluted squander.

Try not to leave or discard squander outside as Monkeypox infection diseases in untamed life might happen.

Expendable creature lodging, dispensable rat bedding, and creature squander that can't be washed away for good ought to be fixed in a pack and discarded appropriately to keep these materials from tainting individuals or different creatures, including wild creatures and family bothers like mice and rodents. Adhere to rules for Disinfecting Home and Other Non-Healthcare Settings.

Bedding, nooks, food dishes, and some other things in direct contact with tainted creatures should be appropriately sanitized following the Disinfecting Home and Other Non-Healthcare Settings.

Dirtied clothing and bedding (counting dispensable rat bedding) ought not to be shaken or on the other hand if not taken care of in a way that might scatter irresistible particles.

# Treatment

There are no medicines explicitly for monkeypox infection diseases. Notwithstanding, monkeypox and smallpox infections are hereditarily comparable, and that implies that antiviral medications and antibodies created to safeguard against smallpox might be utilized to forestall and treat monkeypox infection contaminations.

Antivirals, for example, tecovirimat (TPOXX), might be suggested for individuals who are bound to get seriously sick, similar to patients with debilitated insusceptible frameworks.

Assuming you have side effects of monkeypox, you ought to converse with your medical care supplier, regardless of whether you assume you had contact with somebody who has monkeypox.

## UNITED STATE flare-up 2022 circumstance synopsis

What You Need to Know

CDC is following an episode of monkeypox that has spread across a few nations that don't ordinarily report monkeypox, including the United States.

The monkeypox infection is spreading for the most part through close, personal contact with somebody who has monkeypox.

You can do whatever it may take to forestall getting monkeypox and bring down your menace during sex.

CDC suggests immunization for individuals who have been presented with monkeypox and individuals who are at a higher threat of being presented with monkeypox.

On the off chance that you have any side effects of monkeypox, converse with your medical services supplier, regardless of whether you assume you had contact with somebody who has monkeypox.

CDC is asking medical services suppliers in the United States to be ready for patients who have rash diseases predictable with monkeypox.

## What clinical experts ought to be aware

Clinicians ought to test patients with rash reliable with monkeypox, which includes injuries that are firm or rubbery, very much surrounded, well established, and frequently foster umbilication during the pustular stage.

A few patients present with a febrile prodrome, which could incorporate discomfort, chills, migraine, or lymphadenopathy.

The rash related to monkeypox can be mistaken for different sicknesses that are experienced in clinical practice (e.g., auxiliary syphilis, herpes, chancroid, and varicella zoster).

Most cases in the ongoing flare-up to date have happened among gay, sexually unbiased, and different men who have intercourse with men, and quiet, paying little mind to sexual or orientation personality, with rash reliable with monkeypox ought to consider for the test. Close actual contact with an individual's irresistible sores or respiratory emissions or openness to defiled materials, for example, dress or bedding can bring about transmission.

Clinicians might counsel their nearby wellbeing division for inquiries concerning monkeypox, including testing.

## Interval Clinical Guidance for the Treatment of Monkeypox

Many individuals tainted with monkeypox infection have a gentle, self-restricting illness course without explicit treatment. Be that as it may, the guess for monkeypox relies upon numerous elements, like past immunization status, starting wellbeing status, simultaneous diseases, and comorbidities among others. Patients who ought to be considered for treatment following a meeting with CDC could include:

Individuals with extreme illness (e.g., hemorrhagic infection, blended sores, sepsis, encephalitis, or different circumstances requiring hospitalization)

Individuals who might be at a high risk of extreme illness:

Individuals with immunocompromise (e.g., human immunodeficiency infection/AIDS contamination, leukemia, lymphoma, summed up the danger, strong organ transplantation, treatment with alkylating specialists, antimetabolites, radiation, growth rot factor inhibitors, high-portion corticosteroids, being a beneficiary with hematopoietic immature microorganism relocate <24 months post-relocate or ≥24 months yet with unite versus-have illness or sickness backslide or having immune system infection with immunodeficiency as a clinical part)

1. Pediatric populaces, especially patients more youthful than 8 years old
2. Individuals with a set of experiences or presence of atopic dermatitis, people with other dynamic exfoliative skin conditions (e.g., dermatitis, consumes, impetigo, varicella zoster infection contamination, herpes simplex infection disease, serious skin inflammation, extreme diaper dermatitis

with broad areas of stripped skin, psoriasis, or Darier sickness [keratosis follicularis])
Pregnant or breastfeeding ladies

3. Individuals with at least one inconvenience (e.g., auxiliary bacterial skin contamination; gastroenteritis with serious sickness/heaving, loose bowels, or lack of hydration; bronchopneumonia; simultaneous infection or other comorbidities)
4. Individuals with monkeypox infection deviant diseases that remember unplanned implantation for eyes, mouth, or other physical regions where monkeypox infection contamination could comprise a unique danger (e.g., the private parts or rear-end)

# Clinical Countermeasures Available for the Treatment of Monkeypox

As of now, there is no treatment endorsed explicitly for monkeypox infection diseases. In any case, antivirals created for use in patients with smallpox might demonstrate help against monkeypox. The accompanying clinical countermeasures are presently accessible from the Strategic National Stockpile (SNS) as choices for the treatment of monkeypox:

" People who have skin conditions, and deviant contaminations actuated by vaccinia infection (besides in instances of detached keratitis). CDC holds an extended admittance convention that permits the utilization of VIGIV for the treatment of orthopoxviruses (counting monkeypox) in a flare-up.

Utilization of VIG has no demonstrated advantage in the treatment of monkeypox and it is obscure whether an individual with extreme monkeypox disease will profit from treatment with VIG. Be that as it may, medical services suppliers might think about its utilization in extreme cases.

VIG can be considered for prophylactic use in an uncovered individual with serious immunodeficiency in T-cell capability for which smallpox immunization following openness to monkeypox infection is contraindicated.

Cidofovir (otherwise called Vistide)

Cidofovir is an antiviral prescription that is supported by the FDA, for the treatment of cytomegalovirus (CMV) retinitis in patients with Acquired Immunodeficiency Syndrome (AIDS).

Information isn't accessible on the adequacy of Cidofovir in treating human instances of monkeypox. In any case, it has been demonstrated to be powerful against orthopoxviruses in vitro and in creature studies. CDC holds an extended admittance convention that considers the utilization of stored Cidofovir for the treatment of orthopoxviruses (counting monkeypox) in a flare-up. It is obscure whether an individual with extreme monkeypox contamination will profit from treatment with Cidofovir, even though its utilization might be viewed as in such cases. Brincidofovir might have a better security profile than Cidofovir. Serious renal harmfulness or other unfavorable occasions have not been seen during the treatment of cytomegalovirus diseases with Brincidofovir when contrasted with treatment utilizing Cidofovir.

Immunization Risks and Monkeypox Disease

For most people who have been presented with monkeypox, the dangers of monkeypox illness are more prominent than the dangers from smallpox or monkeypox immunization.

Monkeypox is a serious infection. It causes fever, migraine, muscle throbs, spinal pain, enlarged lymph hubs, a general sensation of distress, depletion, and serious rash. Investigations of monkeypox in Central Africa — where individuals reside in far-off regions and are medicinally underserved — showed that the illness killed up to 11% of individuals tainted.

Interestingly, a great number of people who get smallpox or monkeypox immunization have just minor responses, such as gentle fever, sleepiness, enlarged organs, and redness and tingling where the antibody is given. Be that as it may, these antibodies do have more serious dangers, as well.

In specific gatherings, for example, for individuals with serious safe framework issues, complexities from ACAM2000 can be extreme. If you have worries about whether you ought to get ACAM2000, converse with your medical services supplier. This antibody has the potential for additional secondary effects and unfavorable occasions than the fresher immunization, JYNNEOS.

## CONCLUSION

Observation and fast ID of new cases is basic for flare-up control. During human monkeypox flare-ups, close contact with contaminated people is the main risk factor for monkeypox infection disease. Wellbeing laborers and family individuals are at a more serious menace of the disease. Wellbeing laborers really focusing on patients with thought or affirmed monkeypox infection disease, or taking care of examples from them, ought to execute standard contamination control safety measures. If potential, people recently immunized against smallpox ought to be chosen to really focus on the patient.

www.ingramcontent.com/pod-product-compliance
Lightning Source LLC
LaVergne TN
LVHW050347160826
845677LV00014B/3840

* 9 7 9 8 8 4 5 9 6 7 4 6 6 *